YO-BPY-651

THE NEW GLUCOSE REVOLUTION

Shopper's Guide
to GI Values 2006

ABOUT THE AUTHORS

Jennie Brand-Miller, Ph.D, one of the world's foremost authorities on carbohydrates and the glycemic index, has championed the GI approach to nutrition for more than 20 years. Professor of Nutrition at the University of Sydney and the President of the Nutrition Society of Australia, in 2004 Brand-Miller was awarded Australia's prestigious ATSE Clunies Ross Award for her commitment to advancing science and technology. She is one of the world's most in-demand speakers on the GI and her laboratory at the University of Sydney is the world's foremost GI-testing center.

Kaye Foster-Powell, M. Nutr. & Diet, an accredited dietitian-nutritionist with extensive experience in diabetes management, is the co-author, with Dr. Brand-Miller, of the authoritative tables of GI and glycemic load values published in the *American Journal of Clinical Nutrition*.

A book like this doesn't happen without a great deal of help. We would particularly like to acknowledge and thank Fiona Atkinson and the dedicated GI Testing Team—Anna, Marian and KaiLyn and all our cheerful, well fed volunteers. We would also like to thank Associate Professor Gareth Denyer for his invaluable help with the database.

Other **NEW GLUCOSE REVOLUTION** Titles

THE NEW GLUCOSE REVOLUTION

Shopper's Guide to GI Values 2006

The Authoritative Source of Glycemic Index Values for More than 500 Foods

Dr. Jennie Brand-Miller
and Kaye Foster-Powell

MARLOWE & COMPANY
NEW YORK

THE NEW GLUCOSE REVOLUTION
SHOPPER'S GUIDE TO GI VALUES 2006:
*The Authoritative Guide to the Glycemic Index
Values for More than 500 Foods*

Copyright © 2006 by Jennie Brand-Miller and Kaye Foster-Powell

Published by
Marlowe & Company
An Imprint of Avalon Publishing Group Incorporated
245 West 17th Street, 11th Floor
New York, NY 10011-5300

AVALON
publishing group incorporated

This edition is being published in somewhat different form
in Australia in 2006 by Hodder Australia, an imprint of
Hachette Livre Australia Pty Ltd. This edition is published
by arrangement with Hachette Livre Australia Pty Ltd.

The GI logo is a trademark of the University of Sydney in Australia
and other countries. A food product carrying this logo is nutritious
and has been tested for its GI by an accredited laboratory.

Library of Congress Cataloging-in-Publication data is available.

ISBN: 1-56924-329-8
ISBN-13: 978-1-56924-329-9

9 8 7 6 5 4 3 2

Designed by India Amos, Neuwirth & Associates, Inc.
Printed in Canada

Contents

Understanding the GI

If **you want** to change to a low-GI diet or increase the amount of low-GI food you are already eating, where do you start? Look no further than *The New Glucose Revolution Shopper's Guide to GI Values 2006*. Many foods today that have been tested by accredited laboratories display the authentic GI symbol. That part is easy. But what about other foods? With hundreds of foods—from breads and breakfast bars to fruit juice, fruit, and vegetables—listed alphabetically, plus by category, this book will save you time in the supermarket by directing you to the best low-GI foods available.

And you don't have to worry about giving up some of your favorite snacks or meals. Simply by swapping from one brand or type of food to another, you can improve the overall GI of your diet. This is where the tables in this book will become an essential part of your food shopping forever.

But first, what are the benefits of a low-GI diet? There's no doubt that knowing the GI values of foods is your key to the enormous health benefits of *The New Glucose Revolution*.

Whether you are overweight, have diabetes, hypertension, elevated blood fats, heart disease, or Syndrome X (the metabolic syndrome), you will benefit from eating a low-GI diet. Or, if you want to do what you can to prevent these problems, you need to know about the glycemic index of foods. You may think you already eat a high-quality diet but being aware of the GI values of foods is essential if you are interested in maintaining optimum health.

With that in mind, we've put together this handy guide full of GI values to help you put those low-GI smart carb food choices into your shopping cart and onto your plate. By doing so you'll satisfy your hunger, increase your energy levels, and eliminate your desire to eat more than you should.

How to use the tables:

▶ if you want the actual GI value and glycemic load (GL) of a food, turn to page 35 for a comprehensive A–Z listing of individual foods with their GI and GL.

We have cross-referenced this listing so you can check by brand name, by food type, or by food category.

▶ if you want to know whether a food is high, moderate, or low GI, start on page 77 for our at-a-glance Low GI, Medium GI, and High GI listings

You can use the different listings to:

▶ find the GI of your favorite foods
▶ compare foods within a category (two types of bread, for example)
▶ improve your diet by finding a low-GI substitute for high-GI foods
▶ put together a low-GI meal
▶ shop for low-GI foods

If you can't find the GI value for a food you regularly eat, please write to the manufacturer and encourage them to have the food tested by an accredited laboratory such as Canada's Glycemic Index Laboratories. They can be contacted on the web at *www.gilabs.com* or via email at info

The GI values in this book are correct at the time of publication. However, the formulation of commercial foods can change and the GI may change, too. You can rely on foods showing the GI symbol. Although some manufacturers include the GI value of their product on the label, you would need to know that the testing was carried out independently by an accredited laboratory, as represented by the authentic GI symbol (See page 32.)

THE GI EXPLAINED

Our research on the GI began more than 20 years ago at about the time when health authorities around the world began to stress the importance of high-carbohydrate diets. Until then dietary fat had grabbed all the public and scientific attention, but low-fat diets are by their very nature *automatically* high in carbohydrate. The rapidly rising numbers of people with obesity at this time led nutrition scientists to start asking questions—could carbohydrates be implicated in the development of obesity, are all carbohydrates the same, are all starches good for health and all sugars bad? To investigate, they began to study the effects of carbohydrates on blood glucose levels. They wanted to know which carbohydrate foods were associated with the least fluctuation in blood glucose levels and the best for overall health, including reduced risk of diabetes and heart disease.

Understanding the GI of foods helps you choose the right amount of carbohydrate and the right sort of carbohydrate for your long-term health and well-being. The GI is a physiologically based measure of the effect carbohydrates have on blood glucose levels. It provides an easy and effective way to eat a healthy diet and at the same time control fluctuations in blood glucose.

▶ Carbohydrates that break down quickly during digestion, releasing glucose quickly into the blood stream, have a high GI

▶ Carbohydrates that break down slowly, releasing glucose into the blood stream gradually, have a low GI. We call these smart carbs.

A low-GI diet has been scientifically proven to help people:

▶ with type 1 diabetes
▶ with type 2 diabetes
▶ with gestational diabetes (diabetes during pregnancy)
▶ who are overweight
▶ who have a normal weight but excess abdominal fat
▶ whose blood glucose levels are higher than desirable
▶ who have been told they have prediabetes or are insulin resistant
▶ with high levels of triglycerides and low levels of HDL cholesterol ("good" cholesterol)
▶ with Syndrome X (the insulin resistance or metabolic syndrome)

▶ who suffer from polycystic ovarian syndrome (PCOS)
▶ who suffer from fatty liver disease (NAFLD or NASH)

If you would like to know more about the beneficial effects eating low-GI foods can have on the above conditions, please refer to our other books in *The New Glucose Revolution* series, a full list of which can be found at the beginning of this book.

The rate of carbohydrate digestion has important implications for everybody. For most people, foods with a low GI have advantages over those with a high GI. They can:

▶ improve blood glucose control
▶ increase satiety as they are more filling and satisfying and reduce appetite
▶ facilitate weight loss
▶ improve blood fat profiles
▶ reduce risks of developing diabetes, heart disease, and certain types of cancer

MAKING THE CHANGE
TO A LOW-GI DIET

Three things to remember:

1. The GI relates only to carbohydrate-rich foods

There are three main nutrients in food—protein, carbohydrate, and fat. Meat, chicken, eggs, and fish are high in protein; bread, rice, pasta, and cereals are high in carbohydrate; and butter, margarine, and oils are high in fat. We can only measure the GI of foods that contain carbohydrate.

2. The GI is not intended to be used in isolation

The GI value of a food alone does not make it good or bad for us. It is important to consider the overall nutritional value of a food, including the saturated fat, salt, and fiber content—in addition to its GI value—when choosing foods for a balanced diet.

3. There is no need to eat only low-GI foods

While most of us will benefit from eating low-GI foods at each meal, this doesn't mean consuming these foods to the exclusion of all other carb foods. When we eat a combination of low and high-GI carb foods, like fruit and sandwiches, lentils with rice, potatoes and corn, the final GI value of the meal is intermediate.

To get started, you need to:

EAT a lot more fruit and vegetables, legumes and wholegrain products such as barley and traditional oats.

PAY ATTENTION to breads and breakfast cereals—these food contribute most to the glycemic load of a typical American diet.

MINIMIZE refined flour products and starches such as crackers, cookies, rolls, and pastries, irrespective of their fat and sugar content.

AVOID high-GI snacks such as pretzels, corn chips, rice cakes, and crackers.

SEVEN TOP TIPS FOR EATING THE HEALTHY LOW-GI WAY

1. Eat seven or more servings of fruit and vegetables every day (two fruit and five veggies)

Being high in fiber, and therefore filling, and low in fat (apart from olives and avocado, which contain "good" fats), fruit and vegetables play a central role in low-GI eating. They are bursting with vitamins, minerals, antioxidants, and phytochemicals, which will give you a glow of good health.

2. Eat low-GI breads and cereals

The type of bread and cereals you eat affects the GI of your diet the most. Mixed grain breads, sourdough, traditional rolled oats, bulgur wheat, pearl barley, pasta, noodles, and certain types of rice are just a few examples of low-GI cereal foods.

3. Eat more legumes, including soybeans, chickpeas, and lentils

Whether you buy dried beans, chickpeas, or lentils and cook them yourself at home or opt for the convenient, time-saving canned varieties, you are choosing one of nature's lowest GI foods.

4. Eat nuts in small amounts regularly

Although nuts are high in fat (averaging around 50 percent), it is largely unsaturated fat, so they make a healthy substitute for snacks such as cookies, cakes, pastries, potato chips, and chocolate.

5. Eat more fish and seafood

Increased fish consumption is linked to a reduced risk of coronary heart disease, improvements in mood, lower rates of depression, better blood fat levels, and enhanced immunity.

6. Eat lean red meats, poultry, and eggs

These protein foods do not have a GI because they are not sources of carbohydrate. Red meat, however, is the best source of iron you can get. Good iron status can increase your energy levels and improve your exercise tolerance.

7. Eat low-fat dairy foods

Milk, cheese, ice cream, yogurt, and buttermilk (deleted custard) are the richest sources of calcium in our diet.

YOUR DAILY FOOD CHOICES

Three key habits to ensure a low-GI diet

1. If you eat breakfast cereal, check out the GI of your favorite brand—you might be surprised. Most of the popular big-name cereals have high GI values in the 70s and above.
2. Choose low-GI bread. Steer clear of cookies, cakes, doughnuts, and bread rolls made of refined flour (except sourdough) as much as you can.
3. Eat fruit for at least one of your daily snacks and have a low-fat milk drink or low-fat yogurt for another.

Healthy low-GI diet tips

▶ Focus on what you eat, rather than what not to eat.

▶ Eat at least one low-GI food at each meal.

▶ Reduce your intake of fat, especially saturated.

▶ Eat regularly; don't skip meals.

To help you achieve your *minimum* requirements for energy, protein, vitamins, and minerals we have created two special GI food pyramids—one for Moderate Carb Eaters and one for Big Carb Eaters.

The recommended servings of each food group are shown with each pyramid. If you are a big bread and cereal eater, the GI pyramid for Big Carb Eaters will suit you best.

Either way, the serving information on page 16 applies to both pyramids.

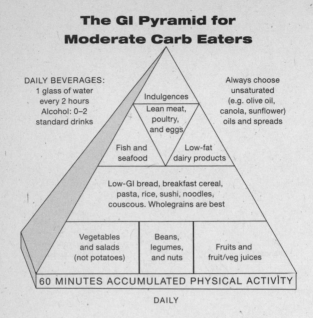

The GI Pyramid for Moderate Carb Eaters

DAILY BEVERAGES:
1 glass of water
every 2 hours
Alcohol: 0–2
standard drinks

Always choose
unsaturated
(e.g. olive oil,
canola, sunflower)
oils and spreads

Indulgences

Lean meat,
poultry,
and eggs

Fish and
seafood

Low-fat
dairy products

Low-GI bread, breakfast cereal,
pasta, rice, sushi, noodles,
couscous. Wholegrains are best

Vegetables
and salads
(not potatoes)

Beans,
legumes,
and nuts

Fruits and
fruit/veg juices

60 MINUTES ACCUMULATED PHYSICAL ACTIVITY

DAILY

Daily food choices for Moderate Carb Eaters:

Indulgences: 1–2 servings

Fish and seafood/lean meat, poultry, and eggs:
5–7 servings

Low-fat dairy products: 2 servings

Bread, breakfast cereals, rice, pasta, noodles, grains:
4 servings

Vegetables and salads: 5 or more servings

Legumes: 1–2 servings

Fruit and juices: 1–3 servings

Nuts and oils: 2–4 servings

The serving guidelines shown above are for the lowest recommended level of carbohydrate intake (40–45% of energy from carbohydrate) for a 1400–1900 calorie diet. For the lower calorie intake, choose the smaller number of servings.

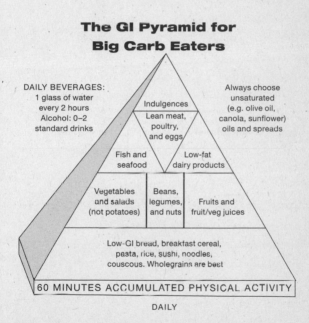

The GI Pyramid for Big Carb Eaters

DAILY BEVERAGES:
1 glass of water every 2 hours
Alcohol: 0–2 standard drinks

Always choose unsaturated (e.g. olive oil, canola, sunflower) oils and spreads

Indulgences

Lean meat, poultry, and eggs

Fish and seafood

Low-fat dairy products

Vegetables and salads (not potatoes)

Beans, legumes, and nuts

Fruits and fruit/veg juices

Low-GI bread, breakfast cereal, pasta, rice, sushi, noodles, couscous. Wholegrains are best

60 MINUTES ACCUMULATED PHYSICAL ACTIVITY

DAILY

Daily food choices for Big Carb Eaters:

Indulgences: 1–2 servings

Fish and seafood/lean meat, poultry, and eggs:
   3–5 servings

Low-fat dairy products: 2 servings

Bread, breakfast cereals, rice, pasta, noodles, grains:
  6–8 servings
Vegetables and salads: 5 or more servings
Legumes: 1–2 servings
Fruit and juices: 3 servings
Nuts and oils: 2–3 servings

The serving guidelines shown above are for an average carbohydrate intake (50–55% of energy from carbohydrate) for a 1400–1900 calorie diet. For the lower calorie intake, choose the smaller number of servings.

What's a serving?

Whether you eat carbs in moderate or large amounts, the portion sizes stay the same.

Indulgences

2 tablespoons cream, sour cream
1 ounce chocolate
1 small slice (about 1½ ounces) cake
1 small bag (1 ounce) potato chips
2 standard alcoholic drinks* (a 5-ounce glass of wine, 1½ ounces of distilled spirits, or a 12-ounce beer)

---

* National guidelines recommend an average daily limit of one standard alcoholic drink for women and two for men.

Fish, seafood, lean meats, poultry, eggs & alternatives

3 ounces (cooked) boneless meat, fish, or chicken

3 ounces canned fish

2 eggs

1½ ounces reduced-fat cheese or 1 ounce full fat cheese

3½ ounces tofu

Legumes

½ cup cooked lentils, chickpeas, beans

Low-fat dairy or alternative

1 cup milk or soy milk

1 cup yogurt

Nuts & oils

2 teaspoons olive or canola oil

1 tablespoon oil-based vinaigrette

½ ounce nuts

¼ cup avocado

Breads, cereals, rice, pasta, noodles, grains

1 slice bread

½ cup cooked rice, pasta, or noodles

½ cup cereal

Fruit & juices

1 medium piece of fruit

1 cup small fruit pieces

½ cup juice

Vegetables

½ cup cooked vegetables

1 cup raw or salad vegetables

WHAT TO KEEP IN YOUR PANTRY

Asian sauces: hoisin, oyster, soy, and fish sauces are a good basic range.

Barley: one of the oldest cultivated cereals, barley is very nutritious and high in soluble fiber. Look for products such as pearl barley to use in soups, stews, and pilafs.

Black pepper: buy freshly ground pepper or grind your own peppercorns.

Bread: low-GI options include grainy, stoneground wholemeal, pumpernickel, sourdough, English-style muffins, flat bread, and pita bread.

Breakfast cereals: these include traditional rolled oats, natural muesli, and low-GI packaged breakfast cereals.

Making sense of food labeling

There's lots of information on food labels these days, but unfortunately, very few people know how to interpret it correctly. Often the claims on the front of the package don't mean quite what you think. Here are some prime examples:

Cholesterol free—Take care, the food may still be high in fat.

Reduced fat—But is it low fat? Compare fat per 100 g between products.

No added sugar—Do you realize it could still raise your blood glucose?

Lite—Light in what? It could mean simply light in color.

To get the hard facts on the nutritional value of a food, look at the Nutrition Information table. Here you'll find the details regarding the fat, calorie, carbohydrate, fiber, and sodium content of the food. Here are the key points to look for:

Calories—This is a measure of how much energy we get from a food. For a healthy diet we need to eat more foods with a low energy density and combine them with smaller amounts of higher energy foods. To assess the energy density look at the kcals per 100 grams. A low energy density is less than 120 kcals /100 g.

Fat—We want a low saturated fat content, ideally less than 20% of the total fat. This means that if the total fat content is 10 g you want saturated fat less than 2 g. Strictly speaking, a food can be labeled as low in saturated fat if it contains less than 1.5 g saturated fat/100 g.

Total carbohydrate—This is the starch plus any naturally occurring and added sugars in the food. (There's no need to look at the sugar figure separately since it's the total carbohydrate that affects your blood glucose level.) You could use this figure if you were monitoring your carbohydrate intake and to calculate the glycemic load (GL) of your serving of the food. The GL = grams of total carbohydrate per serve × GI ÷ 100.

Fiber—Most of us don't eat enough fiber in our diet so it's better to look for high-fiber foods. A high-fiber food contains more than 3 g fiber per serving.

Sodium—This is a measure of the nasty part of salt in our food. Our bodies need some salt but most people consume much more than they need. Canned foods in particular tend to be high in sodium. Check the sodium content per 100 g next time you buy—a low sodium food contains less than 140 mg sodium/100 g.

Bulgur wheat: use it to make tabbouli, or add to vegetable burgers, stuffings, soups, and stews.

Canned evaporated skim milk: this makes an excellent substitution for cream in pasta sauces.

Canned fish: keep a good stock of canned tuna packed in spring water, and canned sardines and salmon.

Canned fruit: have a variety of canned fruit on hand, including peaches, pears, apples, and nectarines—choose the brands labeled with "no added sugar" fruit juice syrup.

Canned vegetables: sweet corn kernels and tomatoes can help to boost the vegetable content of a meal. Tomatoes, in particular, can be used freely because they are rich in antioxidants, as well as having a low GI.

Couscous: ready in minutes, serve with casseroles and braised dishes.

Curry pastes: a tablespoon or so makes a delicious curry base.

Dried fruit: these include apricots, raisins, prunes, and apples.

Dried herbs: oregano, basil, ground coriander, thyme, and rosemary can be useful to have on standby in the pantry.

Honey: try to avoid the commercial honeys or honey blends, and use the "pure" honey, locally harvested, if possible. These varieties have a much lower GI naturally.

Jam: a dollop of good-quality jam (with no added sugar) on toast contains fewer calories than butter or margarine.

Legumes: stock a variety of legumes (dried or canned), including lentils, split peas, and beans. There are many bean varieties, including cannellini, butter, cranberry, kidney, and soy beans.

Mustard: seeded or wholegrain mustard is useful as a sandwich spread, and in salad dressings and sauces.

Noodles: Many Asian noodles such as Hokkien, udon, and rice vermicelli have low to intermediate

GI values because of their dense texture, whether they are made from wheat or rice flour.

Nuts: try a handful of nuts (about 1 ounce) every other day.

Oils: try olive oil for general use; some extra-virgin olive oil for salad dressings, marinades, and dishes that benefit from its flavor; and sesame oil for Asian–style stir-fries. Canola or olive oil cooking sprays are handy too.

Pasta: a great source of carbohydrates and B vitamins.

Quinoa: this whole grain cooks in about 10–15 minutes and has a slightly chewy texture. It can be used as a substitute for rice, couscous, or bulgur wheat. It is very important to rinse the grains thoroughly before cooking.

Rice: Basmati rice or Uncle Ben's Converted long grain rice are good choices because they have a lower GI than, for example, jasmine rice.

Rolled oats: besides their use in oatmeal, oats can be added to cakes, cookies, breads, and desserts.

Sea salt: use in moderation.

Spices: most spices, including ground cumin, turmeric, cinnamon, paprika, and nutmeg, should be bought in small quantities because they lose pungency with age and incorrect storage.

Stock: make your own stock or buy ready-made products, that are available in long-life cartons in the supermarket. To keep the sodium content down with ready-made stocks, look out for a low salt option.

Tomato paste: use in soups, sauces, and casseroles.

Vinegar: white wine or red wine vinegar and balsamic vinegar are excellent as vinaigrette dressings in salads.

WHAT TO KEEP IN YOUR REFRIGERATOR

Bacon: bacon is a valuable ingredient in many dishes because of the flavor it offers. You can make a little bacon go a long way by trimming off all fat and chopping it finely. Lean ham is often a more economical and leaner way to go.

Bottled vegetables: sun-dried tomatoes, olives, grilled eggplant and peppers are handy to keep as flavorful additions to pastas and sandwiches.

Capers, olives, and anchovies: these can be bought in jars and kept in the refrigerator once opened. They are a tasty (but salty) addition to pasta dishes, salads, and pizzas.

Cheese: any reduced-fat cheese is great to keep handy in the fridge. A block of Parmesan is indispensable and will keep for up to a month. Reduced-fat cottage and ricotta cheeses have a short life so are best bought as needed, and they can be a good alternative to butter or margarine in a sandwich.

Condiments: keep jars of minced garlic, chile, or ginger in the refrigerator to spice up your cooking in an instant.

Eggs: to enhance your intake of omega-3 fats, we suggest using omega-3-enriched eggs. Although the yoke is high in cholesterol, the fat in eggs is predominantly monounsaturated, and therefore considered a "good fat."

Fish: try a variety of fresh fish.

Fresh herbs: these are available in most supermarkets and there really is no substitute for the flavor they impart. For variety, try parsley, basil, mint, chives, and coriander.

Fresh fruit Almost all fruits make an excellent low-GI snack. When in season, try fruit such as apples, oranges, pears, grapes, grapefruit, peaches, apricots, strawberries, and mangoes.

Meat: lean varieties are better—try lean beef, lamb fillets, pork fillets, chicken (breast or drumsticks), and ground beef.

Milk: skim or low-fat milk is best, or try low-fat calcium-enriched soy milk.

Vegetables: keep a variety of seasonal vegetables on hand such as spinach, broccoli, cauliflower, Asian greens, asparagus, zucchini, and mushrooms. Peppers, scallions, and sprouts (mung bean and snow-pea sprouts) are great to bulk up a salad. Sweet corn, sweet potato, and yam are essential to your low-GI food store.

Yogurt: low-fat natural yogurt provides the most calcium for the fewest calories. Have vanilla or fruit versions as a dessert, or use natural yogurt as a condiment in savory dishes.

WHAT TO KEEP IN YOUR FREEZER

Frozen berries: berries can make any dessert special, and by using frozen ones it means you don't have to wait until berry season in order to indulge. Try berries such as blueberries, raspberries, and strawberries.

Frozen yogurt: this is a fantastic substitute for ice cream and some products even have a similar creamy texture, but with much less fat.

Frozen vegetables: keep a packet of peas, beans, corn, spinach, or mixed vegetables in the freezer—these are handy to add to a quick meal.

Ice cream: reduced or low-fat ice cream is ideal for a quick dessert, served with fresh fruit.

HOW WE CALCULATE THE GI

As we explained earlier, the GI is simply a ranking of the carbohydrate in foods depending on their immediate effect on blood glucose levels. To make an absolutely fair comparison, all foods are tested following an internationally standardized method. The higher the GI the higher the blood glucose levels after consumption.

> ▶ A high GI value is 70 or more
> ▶ A medium GI value is 56 to 69 inclusive
> ▶ A low GI value is 55 or less

The GI rating of a food must be tested physiologically and only a few centers around the world currently provide a legitimate testing service.

Testing the GI of a food requires a group of eight to ten subjects and knowledge of the food's carbohydrate content. After an overnight fast, each subject consumes a portion of the test food containing a specified amount of carbohydrate (usually 50 grams, but sometimes 25 or even 15 grams). Fingerprick blood samples are taken at 15- to 30-minute intervals over the next two hours. During this time, blood glucose levels rise and fall back to baseline levels. The full extent of glycemia (rise in blood glucose) is assessed by measuring the area under the curve using a computer algorithm. For example, our subject, Lisa, eats a 50-gram carbohydrate portion of barley. Her area under the curve was found to be 60 units.

On three other occasions our subjects must consume the reference food (the same amount of carbohydrate given as pure glucose) to determine their average response to the reference food. Our subject Lisa was found to have an average area of 180 units. Each subject's area under the curve to the test food is then expressed as a percentage of their average after the reference food. Lisa's value is (60/180) × 100 = 30. Hence the GI of barley in Lisa's case is 30. There will be some variation between subjects but if we were to test them again and again, all subjects will tend to move toward the average of the whole group.

Is there an easier way to test the GI of a food? No! The GI is *defined* by its standardized method of testing in human subjects (*in vivo* testing). You may hear about *in vitro* (test tube) methods but these are simple short-cut methods that may or may not reflect the true GI of a food. *In vitro* methods may guide food manufacturers during re-formulation of their product, but only *in vivo* testing can give us a GI value.

In the following tables we have also included some foods that contain very little carbohydrate or none at all because so many people ask us for their GI. Many vegetables such as avocado and broccoli, and protein-rich foods such as eggs, cheese, chicken, and tuna are among the low or no carbohydrate category. We show this as ★. Most alcoholic beverages are also low in carbohydrate.

LET'S TALK
GLYCEMIC LOAD (GL)

In addition to the GI values, the tables in this book include the GL (glycemic load) of normal-sized portions of the food on your plate. Glycemic load is the product of GI and the amount of carbohydrate in a serving of food. You can think about GL as the amount of carbohydrate "adjusted" for its GI. This means that you can choose foods with either a low GI and/or a low GL.

When we eat a meal containing carbohydrate, our blood glucose rises and falls. The extent to which it rises and remains high is critically important to health and depends on two things: the amount of carbohydrate in the meal and the nature of that carbohydrate (its GI value). Both are equally important determinants of changes in blood glucose levels.

Researchers at Harvard University came up with a way of combining and describing these two factors with the term "glycemic load." The glycemic load helps us predict what the effect of a particular carbohydrate food will be on our blood glucose level after consuming that food. The glycemic load is greatest for high-GI foods containing the most carbohydrate (such as rice or bread), especially when eaten in large quantities.

Don't get carried away with glycemic load. The glycemic load doesn't distinguish "slow carbs" from "low carbs." It is much better to make food choices based on the GI rather than the GL because you want to see at least moderate amounts of carbohydrates in your meal. If you choose only on the basis of glycemic load, you could easily find yourself eating a lot of unwanted fat and excess protein. Low-GI carbohydrates give you much more than just control of blood glucose—you'll feel fuller for longer thanks to prolonged absorption and you'll reduce your insulin levels at the same time.

The glycemic load is calculated simply by multiplying the GI value of a food by the amount of carbohydrate per serving and dividing by 100.

Glycemic load (GL) =
(GI value × carbohydrate per serving) ÷ 100

For example, an apple has a GI value of 40 and contains 15 grams of carbohydrate per serving. Its GL is:

$$(40 \times 15) \div 100 = 6.$$

A potato has a GI value of 90 and 20 grams of carbohydrate per serving. It has a GL of:

$$(90 \times 20) \div 100 = 18.$$

This is not to say that the glycemic response will be

exactly three times higher for a potato compared with an apple, but the total metabolic effect, including overall insulin demand, might be three times higher.

Don't use the GL values in isolation!

If you use GL values alone, you might find yourself eating a diet with *very little carbohydrate* and a whole heap of fat, especially saturated fat, and excessive amounts of protein! GL does not distinguish between "**low** carb" and "**slow** carb."

So what should you do?

▶ Use the GI to compare foods of a similar nature (breads with breads); **The low-GI varieties will have the lower GL values.**
▶ Use the GL when comparing foods with a high GI but low carbohydrate content per serving.

Remember that the GL values listed in the following tables are for the specified nominal portion size. If you eat more (or less) you will need to calculate another GL value.

> Low GL = 10 or less
> Medium GL = 11–19
> High GL = 20 or more

LOOK FOR THE AUTHENTIC GI SYMBOL ON FOODS

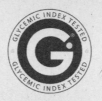

This symbol on food packaging is your guarantee that the product has had its GI tested accurately (by an accredited laboratory) and meets strict nutritional criteria. The food packaging will clearly indicate if a food is high, medium, or low GI. Whether high, medium, or low GI, you can be assured that these foods are healthier choices within their food group, and will make a nutritious contribution to your diet. And it allows you, the consumer, to make an informed choice as to how you balance your overall diet.

The GI Symbol Program was established by the University of Sydney, Diabetes Australia, and the Juvenile Diabetes Research Foundation whose expertise in GI is recognized internationally. The Program is committed to a global vision of healthier populations through nutritionally-balanced lower GI diets.

So, for healthier lifestyle choices you can trust, look for the authentic GI symbol when you're shopping. For more information and the latest list of approved products, visit us at: **www.gisymbol.com**

Things you should know about the GI Symbol

▶ Foods that carry the certification mark are healthy in many respects. To be eligible, foods must meet other strict nutrient criteria relating to carbohydrate, total fat, salt, calories, and be a good source of fiber.

▶ Manufacturers pay a license fee to use the certification mark on their products. The fee is paid to GI Limited, a non-profit partnership between the University of Sydney, Diabetes Australia, and the Juvenile Diabetes Research Foundation. The fee helps to fund sensible, balanced communication about the GI, healthy eating, and research.

▶ High-GI foods can carry the symbol. Remember, you don't need to eat low GI all the time—an informed person can mix and match as he or she sees fit.

▶ If you have type 1 diabetes, you may need to consider the quantity of carbohydrate in each serving of food, in addition to the GI. Calculating the GL (GI × carbohydrate per serving/100) is one way of estimating the total glycemic effect.

▶ A food may be reliably tested and not carry the certification mark. It's the manufacturer's choice, but as a consumer you may find it hard to distinguish between reliable and unreliable claims. Look for the GI symbol as your trusted signpost to healthier foods.

A to Z
GI Values

*C*onsult these tables when you want to locate the GI value of a popular food quickly. Here foods are listed alphabetically—both on an individual basis and within their specific food category.

Food category entries include:

Key

★ Means that a food has such a low carbohydrate content that the GI cannot be
measured. See page 27 for more details
on measuring a food's GI.

■ Means that a food may be high in saturated
fat. As we have mentioned previously, the
GI should not be used in isolation, but the
overall nutritional value of the food needs
to be considered.

ⓖ Means that a food has been accurately
tested for its GI *and* meets strict nutritional
criteria. You can be assured that these
foods are healthier choices within their food
categories.

Food	GI	Nominal Serving Size	Available Carbs per Serving	GL per Serving
Alfalfa sprouts, raw	★	½ cup	0	0
All-Bran®, breakfast cereal, Kellogg's®	34	½ cup	15	4
Angel food cake, plain	67 ■	⅛ cake (2 ounces)	29	19
APPLE JUICE				
Apple and blackcurrant juice, unsweetened	45	8 fluid ounces	21	10
Apple and cherry juice, unsweetened Ⓖ	43	8 fluid ounces	33	14
Apple and mango juice, unsweetened Ⓖ	47	8 fluid ounces	27	12
Apple juice, clear, no added sugar Ⓖ	44	8 fluid ounces	30	13
Apple juice, cloudy, no added sugar Ⓖ	37	8 fluid ounces	28	10
Apple muffin, homemade	46 ■	1 small (2 ounces)	29	13
Apple, dried	29	2 ounces	34	10
Apple, fresh	38	1 small (4 ounces)	15	6
Apricot fruit spread, reduced-sugar	55	2 Tbsp.	13	7
Apricot-filled fruit bar, made with whole grain flour	50 ■	1.75 ounces	34	17
Apricots, canned in light syrup	64	½ cup	19	12
Apricots, dried	30	2 ounces	28	9
Apricots, fresh	57	3 small (6 ounces)	13	7
Arborio risotto rice, white, boiled	69	¾ cup	43	29
Arrowroot biscuits	69 ■	1 ounce	18	12

Food	GI	Nominal Serving Size	Available Carbs per Serving	GL per Serving
Artichokes, globe, fresh or canned	★	½ cup	0	0
Arugula, raw	★	1 cup	0	0
Asparagus	★	½ cup	0	0
Avocado	★	2 Tbsp.	0	0
Bacon, lean	★	2 medium strips (½ ounce)	0	0
Bagel, white	72	1 small (2.5 ounces)	35	25
Baked beans, canned in tomato sauce, Heinz®	49	½ cup	17	8
Banana bread, home-made	51 ■	1 slice (3 ounces)	38	18
Banana smoothie, soy drink, low-fat	30	8 fluid ounces	22	7
Banana, ripe	52	1 small (4 ounces)	26	13
Barley, pearled, boiled	25	1 cup	32	8
Basmati rice, white, boiled	58	1 cup	38	22
Bean sprouts	★	½ cup	0	0
BEANS/LEGUMES				
Baked beans, canned in tomato sauce, Heinz®	49	½ cup	17	8
Black beans, boiled	30	¾ cup	25	5
Black-eyed peas, boiled	42	¾ cup	29	12
Butter beans, boiled	31	½ cup	20	6
Cannellini beans, canned	31	½ cup	12	4
Chickpeas, canned	40	½ cup	22	9
Kidney beans, dark red, canned, drained	43	½ cup	25	7
Kidney beans, red, canned, drained	36	½ cup	17	9

Food	GI	Nominal Serving Size	Available Carbs per Serving	GL per Serving
BEANS/LEGUMES (*continued*)				
Lentils, green or brown, dried, boiled	30	¾ cup	17	5
Lentils, red, dried, boiled	26	¾ cup	18	5
Lima beans, baby, frozen, reheated	32	½ cup	30	10
Mung beans	39	½ cup	17	5
Soybeans, canned, drained	14	½ cup	6	1
Split peas, yellow, boiled	32	¾ cup	19	6
White beans, canned	38	½ cup	31	12
Beef, ground, lean	★ ■	3 ounces	0	0
Beef pot pie, with crust	45 ■	3.5 ounces	27	12
Beer (4.6% alcohol)	66	8 fluid ounces	10	0
Beets, red, canned	64	½ cup	7	5
BEVERAGES				
Coffee, black, no milk or sugar	★	8 fluid ounces	0	0
Ensure™, vanilla, nutritional supplement	48	8 fluid ounces	34	16
Malted milk powder in reduced-fat milk	40	8 fluid ounces	31	12
Malted milk powder in skim milk	46	8 fluid ounces	24	11
Malted milk powder in whole milk	45 ■	8 fluid ounces	24	11
Nestle Quik® powder, Chocolate, in reduced-fat milk	41	8 fluid ounces	11	5
Nestle Quik® powder, Strawberry, in reduced-fat milk	35	8 fluid ounces	12	4

Food	GI	Nominal Serving Size	Available Carbs per Serving	GL per Serving
Slim-Fast® drink powder, all flavors, made with skim milk	35	8 fluid ounces	34	12
Slim-Fast® drink, can, vanilla or chocolate	39	8 fluid ounces	39	15
Black bean soup, canned	64	1 cup	27	17
Black beans, boiled	30	¾ cup	25	5
Black-eyed peas, boiled	42	¾ cup	29	12
Blueberry muffin, commercially-made	59 ■	1 small (2 ounces)	29	17
Bok choy	★	½ cup	0	0
Bran Flakes™, breakfast cereal, Kellogg's®	74	¾ cup	18	13
Bran muffin, commercially-made	60 ■	1 small (2 ounces)	24	15
BREAD				
9 Grain mutigrain bread Ⓖ	43	1 slice	14	6
Bagel, white	72	1 small (2.5 ounces)	35	25
Dinner roll, white	73	1 small (1 ounce)	16	12
Flaxseed and soy bread	55	1 slice	24	13
Gluten-free, multigrain bread	79	1 slice	13	10
Hamburger bun, white	61	½ bun (1 ounce)	15	9
Kaiser roll, white	73	½ roll (1 ounce)	16	12
Oat bran and honey bread Ⓖ	49	1 slice	13	7
Pita bread, 4", white	57	1 pita	17	10
Pumpernickel bread	50	1 slice	10	5

Food	GI	Nominal Serving Size	Available Carbs per Serving	GL per Serving
BREAD *(continued)*				
Raisin bread	63	1 slice	17	11
Rye bread, black	76	1 slice	13	10
Rye bread, dark	86	1 slice	14	12
Rye bread, light	68	1 slice	14	10
Rye bread, seeded Ⓖ	51	1 slice	13	7
Sourdough rye bread	48	1 slice	12	6
Sourdough wheat bread	54	1 slice	14	8
Spelt multigrain bread	54	1 slice	12	7
Stuffing, bread	74	½ cup	21	16
Sunflower and barley bread	57	1 slice	11	6
White bread, enriched, sliced	71	1 slice	14	10
Whole wheat bread, made w/enriched wheat flour, sliced	71	1 slice	12	9
Whole wheat bread, 100%, stoneground	59	1 slice	12	7
Wonder White®, bread, sliced	80	1 slice	15	12
BREAKFAST CEREALS				
All-Bran®, Kellogg's®	34	½ cup	15	5
Bran Flakes, Kellogg's®	74	¾ cup	18	13
Coco Pops®, Kellogg's®	77	1 cup	26	20
Corn Flakes®, Kellogg's®	77	1 cup	25	20
Corn Pops®, Kellogg's®	80	1 cup	26	21
Crispix®	87	1 cup	25	22
Froot Loops®, Kellogg's®	69	1 cup	26	18
Frosted Flakes®, Kellogg's®	55	¾ cup	26	15
Honey Smacks®, Kellogg's®	71	1 cup	23	16

Food	GI	Nominal Serving Size	Available Carbs per Serving	GL per Serving
Just Right®, Kellogg's®	60	¾ cup	22	13
Muesli, natural	40	¼ cup	18	8
Muesli, Swiss Formula	56	¼ cup	16	9
Muesli, toasted	43	¼ cup	17	7
Nutri-Grain™, Kellogg's®	66	½ cup	15	10
Oat bran, raw, unprocessed	55	2 Tbsp.	5	3
Oatmeal, instant, made with water	82	1 cup	26	17
Oatmeal, from old-fashioned oats, made with water	60	1 cup	21	11
Oatmeal, from steel-cut oats, made with water	52	1 cup	22	11
Puffed rice	80	2 cups	21	17
Puffed wheat	80	2 cups	21	17
Rice bran, unprocessed	19	4 Tbsp.	14	3
Raisin Bran™, Kellogg's®	73	½ cup	19	14
Rice Krisples®, Kellogg's®	82	1¼ cups	26	22
Semolina, wheat, hot cereal, made with water	55	⅔ cup	11	6
Shredded Wheat	75	½ cup	20	15
Special K®, Kellogg's®	56	1 cup	21	11
Weet-Bix, biscuits, regular	69	½ cup	17	12
Broad beans	79	½ cup	11	9
Broccoli	★	½ cup	0	0
Brown rice, boiled	66	1 cup	37	24
Brussels sprouts	★	½ cup	0	0
Buckwheat pancakes, 6", gluten-free, from pancake mix	102	1 pancake	22	22

Food	GI	Nominal Serving Size	Available Carbs per Serving	GL per Serving
Buckwheat, groats, boiled	54	¾ cup	30	16
Bulghur, cracked wheat, ready to eat	48	½ cup	26	12
Butter beans, boiled	31	½ cup	20	6
Cabbage	★	½ cup	0	0
Cadbury's® Milk Chocolate, plain	49 ■	1 ounce	17	8
CAKES				
Angel food cake, plain	67 ■	⅛ cake (2 ounces)	29	19
Banana bread, home-made	51 ■	1 slice (3 ounces)	38	18
Chocolate cake, cake mix with frosting, Betty Crocker	38 ■	1/12 cake (3.5 ounces)	52	20
Cupcake with strawberry icing	73 ■	1 small (1.5 ounces)	26	19
Pound cake, plain, Sara Lee	54 ■	1 slice (1.75 ounces)	23	12
Sponge cake, plain, unfilled	46 ■	⅛ cake (2 ounces)	36	17
Vanilla cake, cake mix with vanilla frosting, Betty Crocker	42 ■	1/12 cake (3.5 ounces)	58	24
Calamari rings, squid, plain, without batter or breading	★	3 ounces	0	0
Cannellini beans, canned	31	½ cup	12	4
Cantaloupe	67	½ cup	6	4
Capellini, white, boiled	45	1 cup	45	20
Carrot juice, freshly made	43	8 fluid ounces	23	10
Carrot muffin, commercially-made	62 ■	1 small (2 ounces)	32	20

Food	GI	Nominal Serving Size	Available Carbs per Serving	GL per Serving
Carrots, cooked	41	½ cup	5	2
Cashew nuts, salted	22	1 ounce	9	2
Cauliflower	★	½ cup	0	0
Celery	★	½ cup	0	0
CEREAL GRAINS				
Barley, pearled, boiled	25	1 cup	32	8
Buckwheat, groats, boiled	54	¾ cup	30	16
Bulgur, cracked wheat, ready to eat	48	½ cup	26	12
Cornmeal (polenta), cooked with water	68	⅔ cup	13	9
Couscous, boiled	65	1 cup	33	21
Millet, boiled	71	¾ cup	36	25
Cheese	★ ■	1 ounce	0	0
Cheese curls, cheese-flavored snack	74 ■	1.75 ounces	29	22
Cheese tortellini, cooked	50 ■	6 ounces	21	10
Cherries, dark, raw	63	1 cup	12	3
Chicken, without the skin and bone	★ ■	3 ounces	0	0
Chicken nuggets, frozen, reheated	46 ■	3.5 ounces	16	7
Chickpeas, canned	40	½ cup	22	9
Chilies, fresh or dried	★	2 Tbsp.	0	0
Chives, fresh	★	2 Tbsp.	0	0
CHOCOLATE				
Cadbury's® Milk Chocolate, plain	49 ■	1 ounce	17	8
Chocolate cake, cake mix with frosting, Betty Crocker	38 ■	1/12 cake (3 ounces)	52	20

Food	GI	Nominal Serving Size	Available Carbs per Serving	GL per Serving
CHOCOLATE *(continued)*				
Chocolate pudding, instant, package mix, with whole milk	47 ■	½ cup	16	7
Dark chocolate, plain	41 ■	1 ounce	19	8
Dove®, milk chocolate	45 ■	1.5 ounces	29	13
M&M's®, peanut	33 ■	1 ounce	17	6
Mars Bar®, regular	62 ■	2 ounces	40	25
Milk chocolate, plain, with fructose instead of sugar	20 ■	1 ounce	19	4
Nestle®, milk chocolate bar	40	2 ounces	29	12
Snickers Bar®, regular	41 ■	2 ounces	36	15
Twix® bar	44 ■	2 ounces	39	17
White chocolate, plain	44 ■	1.75 ounces	29	13
Clams, plain, steamed	★	3 ounces	0	0
Coca-Cola®, soft drink	53	8 fluid ounces	26	14
Coco Pops®, breakfast cereal, Kellogg's®	77	1 cup	26	20
Coffee, black, no milk or sugar	★	8 fluid ounces	0	0
Condensed milk, sweetened, full-fat	61 ■	2 ounces	28	17
Consommé, clear, chicken or vegetable	★	7 ounces	2	0
COOKIES				
Arrowroot biscuits	69 ■	1 ounce	18	12
Digestives®, cookies, plain	59 ■	1 ounce	16	10
Gluten-free chocolate-coated cookie	35	1 ounce	14	5
Graham crackers, plain	77 ■	1 ounce	18	14

Food	GI	Nominal Serving Size	Available Carbs per Serving	GL per Serving
Oatmeal cookies, plain	54 ■	2 cookies (1 ounce)	17	9
Rich Tea Biscuits®	55 ■	1 ounce	19	10
Shortbread, plain	64 ■	2 cookies (1 ounce)	16	10
Vanilla wafer, plain	77 ■	7 small wafers (1 ounce)	18	14
Corn chips, plain, salted	42 ■	1.75 ounces	25	11
Corn Flakes®, breakfast cereal, Kellogg's®	77	1 cup	25	20
Corn pasta, gluten-free, boiled	78	1¼ cups	42	32
Corn Pops®, breakfast cereal, Kellogg's®	80	1 cup	26	21
Corn, sweet, on the cob	48	1 medium ear	16	8
Corn, sweet, whole kernel, canned	46	⅓ cup	14	7
Cornmeal (polenta), cooked with water	68	⅔ cup	13	9
Couscous, boiled	65	1 cup	33	21
Crabmeat, plain, without breading	★	3 ounces	0	0
CRACKERS AND CRISPBREADS				
Melba toast, plain	70	1 ounce	23	16
Ryvita® Original Rye crispbread	65	1 ounce	30	19
Ryvita® Sesame Original crispbread	64	1 ounce	28	18
Rice cakes, white	82	1 ounce	21	17
Stoned Wheat Thins®	67	1 ounce	17	12
Water crackers, plain	78	1 ounce	18	14

Food	GI	Nominal Serving Size	Available Carbs per Serving	GL per Serving
Cranberries, dried, sweetened	64	1.5 ounces	29	19
Cranberry Juice Cocktail, Ocean Spray®	52	8 fluid ounces	31	16
Crispix®, breakfast cereal	87	1 cup	25	22
Croissant, plain	67 ■	2 ounces	26	17
Cucumber	★	½ cup	0	0
Cupcake, strawberry-iced	73 ■	1 small (1.5 ounces)	26	19
Custard apple, fresh	54	1 small (4 ounces)	19	10
Custard, traditional, homemade	43 ■	½ cup	17	7
Custard, vanilla, reduced fat	37	½ cup	15	6
Dark chocolate, plain	41 ■	1 ounce	19	8
Dates, dried	39	2 ounces	40	16
Diet soft drinks	★	8 fluid ounces	0	0
Digestives® cookies, plain	59 ■	1 ounce	16	10
Dove®, milk chocolate	45 ■	1.5 ounces	29	13
Duck, without the skin and bone	★ ■	3 ounces	0	0
Eggplant	★	½ cup	0	0
Eggs	★ ■	2 eggs	0	0
Endive	★	1 cup	0	0
Ensure™, vanilla, nutritional supplement	48	8 fluid ounces	34	16
Fanta®, orange soft drink	68	8 fluid ounces	34	23
Fennel	★	½ cup	0	0
Fettuccine, egg noodle, cooked	40	1 cup	46	18
Figs, dried	61	2 ounces	26	16

Food	GI	Nominal Serving Size	Available Carbs per Serving	GL per Serving
FISH				
Fish, all-types, fresh or frozen, without skin	★	3 ounces	0	0
Fish sticks, lightly breaded	38 ■	3.5 ounces	19	7
Salmon, canned in water	★	3 ounces	0	0
Sardines, canned	★	2 ounces	0	0
Tuna, canned in water	★	3 ounces	0	0
Flaxseed and soy bread	55	1 slice	24	13
French fries, frozen, reheated	75 ■	5 ounces	29	22
Froot Loops®, breakfast cereal, Kellogg's®	69	1 cup	26	18
Frosted Flakes®, breakfast cereal, Kellogg's®	55	¾ cup	26	15
Fructose, pure	19	1 Tbsp.	10	2
FRUIT AND VEGETABLE JUICE				
Apple and blackcurrant, unsweetened	45	8 fluid ounces	21	10
Apple and cherry, unsweetened Ⓖ	43	8 fluid ounces	33	14
Apple and mango, unsweetened Ⓖ	47	8 fluid ounces	27	12
Apple juice, clear, no added sugar Ⓖ	44	8 fluid ounces	30	13
Apple juice, cloudy, no added sugar Ⓖ	37	8 fluid ounces	28	10
Carrot, freshly made	43	8 fluid ounces	23	10
Cranberry Juice Cocktail, Ocean Spray®	52	8 fluid ounces	31	16
Grapefruit, unsweetened	48	8 fluid ounces	22	9
Orange, unsweetened, fresh	50	8 fluid ounces	18	9

Food	GI	Nominal Serving Size	Available Carbs per Serving	GL per Serving
FRUIT AND VEGETABLE JUICE *(continued)*				
Orange, unsweetened, from concentrate	53	8 fluid ounces	18	9
Pineapple, unsweetened	46	8 fluid ounces	34	16
Prune, unsweetened	43	8 fluid ounces	30	13
Tomato, no added sugar	38	8 fluid ounces	9	4
FRUIT, CANNED				
Apricots, in light syrup	64	½ cup	19	12
Fruit cocktail, in natural juice	55	½ cup	16	9
Lychees, in syrup, drained	79	½ cup	20	16
Peaches, in heavy syrup	58	½ cup	15	9
Peaches, in light syrup	57	½ cup	18	9
Peaches, in natural juice	45	½ cup	11	4
Pear halves, in light syrup	25	½ cup	14	4
Pears, in natural juice	44	½ cup	13	5
FRUIT, DRIED				
Apple	29	2 ounces	34	10
Apricots	30	2 ounces	28	9
Cranberries, sweetened	64	1.5 ounces	29	19
Dates, pitted	103	2 ounces	40	42
Figs, dried	61	2 ounces	26	16
Prunes, pitted, Sunsweet®	29	2 ounces	33	10
Raisins	64	2 ounces	44	28
FRUIT, FRESH				
Apple	38	1 small (4 ounces)	15	6
Apricots	57	3 small (6 ounces)	13	7
Banana, ripe	52	1 small (4 ounces)	26	13

Food	GI	Nominal Serving Size	Available Carbs per Serving	GL per Serving
Canteloupe	67	½ cup	6	4
Cherries, dark	63	1 cup	12	3
Custard apple	54	1 small (4 ounces)	19	10
Grapefruit	25	½ large	11	3
Grapes	53	1 cup	18	8
Kiwi fruit	53	1 medium (4 ounces)	12	6
Lemon	★	1 small	0	0
Lime	★	1 small	0	0
Mango	51	½ medium (4 ounces)	17	8
Montmorency Frozen Tart Cherries	54	½ cup	6	3
Orange	42	1 small (4 ounces)	11	5
Papaya	56	½ small (4 ounces)	8	5
Peach	42	1 medium (4 ounces)	11	5
Pear	38	1 medium (4 ounces)	11	4
Pineapple	59	¾ cup	10	6
Plum	39	1 medium (4 ounces)	12	5
Raspberries	★	½ cup	0	0
Rhubarb	★	1 cup	0	0
Strawberries	40	1 cup	3	1
Watermelon	76	¾ cup	6	4
Garlic	★	1 clove	0	0
Gatorade® sports drink	78	8 fluid ounces	15	12
Gelati, sugar-free, chocolate	37	1 cup	27	10
Gelati, sugar-free, vanilla	39	1 cup	27	11

Food	GI	Nominal Serving Size	Available Carbs per Serving	GL per Serving
Ginger, grated	★	1 tsp.	0	0
GLUTEN-FREE PRODUCTS				
Gluten-free buckwheat pancakes, 6", from pancake mix	102	1 pancake	22	22
Gluten-free chocolate-coated cookie	35	1 ounce	14	5
Gluten-free corn pasta, cooked	78	1¼ cups	42	32
Gluten-free multigrain bread	79	1 slice	13	10
Gluten-free rice and corn pasta, cooked	76	1¼ cups	49	37
Glutinous rice, white, cooked	98	¾ cup	32	31
Gnocchi, cooked	68	6 ounces	48	33
Golden syrup	63	1 Tbsp.	17	11
Graham crackers, plain	77 ■	1 ounce	18	14
Grapefruit juice, unsweetened	48	8 fluid ounces	22	9
Grapefruit, fresh	25	½ large	11	3
Grape jelly Ⓖ	52	1 Tbsp	10	5
Grapes, fresh	53	1 cup	18	8
Green beans	★	½ cup	0	0
Green pea soup, canned	66	8 fluid ounces	41	27
Gummi confectionery, made with glucose syrup	94	1.75 ounces	36	34
Ham, lean	★ ■	3 ounces	0	0
Hamburger bun, white	61	½ bun (1 ounce)	15	9
Herbs, fresh or dried	★	2 Tbsp.	0	0
HONEY				
Honey, commercial-blend	64	1 Tbsp.	17	11

Food	GI	Nominal Serving Size	Available Carbs per Serving	GL per Serving
Honey, 100% pure floral	35	1 Tbsp.	18	6
Honey, various (averaged)	55	1 Tbsp.	18	10
Honey Smacks®, breakfast cereal, Kellogg's	71	1 cup	23	16
Hummus, regular	6	2 Tbsp.	5	1
ICE CREAM				
Gelati, sugar-free, chocolate	37	1 cup	27	10
Gelati, sugar-free, vanilla	39	1 cup	27	11
Ice cream, low-fat, chocolate Ⓖ	49	½ cup	14	7
Ice cream, low-fat, vanilla Ⓖ	46	½ cup	6	3
Ice cream, full-fat, chocolate ■	37 ■	½ cup	9	4
Ice cream, full-fat, vanilla	47 ■	½ cup	15	8
Instant noodles, 99% fat free, dry, package	67	2.5 ounces	51	34
Instant rice, white, boiled	87	¾ cup	42	29
JAM				
Jam, Apricot, 100% fruit	50	1½ Tbsp.	9	4.5
Jam, Blackberry, 100% fruit	46	1½ Tbsp.	9	4
Jam, Raspberry, 100% fruit	46	1½ Tbsp.	9	4
Jam, Strawberry, 100% fruit	46	1½ Tbsp.	9	4
Jasmine rice, white, long-grain	109	¾ cup	42	46
Jelly beans	78	1 ounce	28	22
Jelly, diet	★	2 Tbsp.	0	0

Food	GI	Nominal Serving Size	Available Carbs per Serving	GL per Serving
Jelly, grape Ⓖ	52	1 Tbsp	10	5
Just Right® Just Grains, breakfast cereal, Kellogg's®	62	¾ cup	23	14
Kaiser roll, white	73	½ roll (1 ounce)	16	12
Kidney beans, dark red, canned, drained	43	½ cup	25	7
Kidney beans, red, canned, drained	36	½ cup	17	9
Kiwi fruit, fresh	53	1 medium (4 ounces)	12	6
Lamb, lean	★	3 ounces	0	0
Lean Cuisine®, French-style Chicken with Rice	36	14 ounces	72	26
Leeks	★	½ cup	0	0
Lettuce	★	1 cup	0	0
Licorice, soft	78	2 ounces	42	33
Life Savers®, peppermint	70	1 ounce	30	21
Lima beans, baby, frozen, reheated	32	½ cup	30	10
Lime	★	1 small	0	0
LINGUINE				
Linguine, thick, durum wheat, cooked	46	1 cup	48	22
Linguine, thin, durum wheat, cooked	52	1 cup	45	23
Lobster, plain	★	3 ounces	0	0
Long-grain rice, white, boiled	50	¾ cup	41	23
Lychees, canned, in syrup, drained	79	½ cup	20	16
M&M's®, peanut	33 ■	1 ounce	17	6

Food	GI	Nominal Serving Size	Available Carbs per Serving	GL per Serving
MACARONI				
Macaroni and cheese, Kraft®	64 ■	1¼ cups	51	32
Macaroni, white, durum wheat, cooked	47	1¼ cups	48	23
Macaroni, white, plain, cooked	47	1¼ cups	48	23
Malted milk powder in reduced-fat milk	40	8 fluid ounces	31	12
Malted milk powder in skim milk	46	8 fluid ounces	24	11
Malted milk powder in whole milk	45 ■	8 fluid ounces	24	11
Mango, fresh	51	½ medium (4 ounces)	17	8
MAPLE SYRUP				
Maple syrup, pure, Canadian	54	1 Tbsp.	18	10
Maple-flavored syrup	68	1 Tbsp.	22	15
Marmalade, orange	55	1½ Tbsp.	20	9
Mars Bar®, regular	62 ■	2 ounces	40	25
Marshmallows, plain, white	62	1 ounce	20	12
MEAT				
Bacon, lean	★	2 medium strips (½ ounce)	0	0
Beef, ground, lean	★ ■	3 ounces	0	0
Beef pot pie, with crust	45 ■	3.5 ounces	27	12
Beef, steak, lean	★ ■	3 ounces	0	0
Ham, lean	★ ■	3 ounces	0	0
Lamb, lean	★	3 ounces	0	0
Pork	★ ■	3 ounces	0	0
Salami	★ ■	1 ounce	0	0
Veal	★	3 ounces	0	0

Food	GI	Nominal Serving Size	Available Carbs per Serving	GL per Serving
Melba toast, plain	70	1 ounce	23	16
MILK				
Milk, 1%, light, low-fat	32	8 fluid ounces	12	4
Milk, 2%, reduced-fat	30	8 fluid ounces	14	4
Milk, fat free, skim, nonfat	32	8 fluid ounces	12	4
Milk, whole, full-fat	27 ■	8 fluid ounces	12	4
Milk, low-fat, chocolate, with aspartame	24	8 fluid ounces	15	3
Milk, low-fat, chocolate, with sugar	34	8 fluid ounces	26	9
Condensed milk, sweetened, full-fat	61 ■	2 fluid ounces	28	17
Rice milk, average	92	8 fluid ounces	34	31
Rice milk, calcium-enriched Vitasoy®	79	8 fluid ounces	22	17
Soy milk, full-fat, calcium-fortified	36	8 fluid ounces	18	6
Soy milk, reduced-fat, calcium-fortified	44	8 fluid ounces	17	8
Milk chocolate, plain, with fructose instead of regular sugar	20 ■	1 ounce	19	4
Millet, boiled	71	¾ cup	36	25
Minestrone soup, traditional, canned	39	9 ounces	18	7
MUESLI				
Muesli, natural	40	¼ cup	18	8
Muesli, Swiss Formula	56	¼ cup	16	9
Muesli, toasted	43	¼ cup	17	7

Food	GI	Nominal Serving Size	Available Carbs per Serving	GL per Serving
Muesli bar, chewy, with choc chips or fruit	54 ■	1 ounce	21	12
Muesli bar, crunchy, with dried fruit	61	1 ounce	21	13
MUFFINS				
Apple muffin, home-made	46 ■	1 small (2 ounces)	29	13
Blueberry muffin, commercially-made	59 ■	1 small (2 ounces)	29	17
Bran muffin, commercially-made	60 ■	1 small (2 ounces)	24	15
Carrot muffin, commercially-made	62 ■	1 small (2 ounces)	32	20
Mung bean noodles, cooked	33	1¼ cups	45	18
Mung beans	39	½ cup	17	5
Mushrooms	★	½ cup	0	0
Nestle®, milk chocolate bar	40	2 ounces	29	12
NOODLES				
Instant noodles, 99% fat free, dry, package	67	2.5 ounces	51	34
Mung bean noodles, cooked	33	1¼ cups	45	18
Rice vermicelli, cooked	58	1¼ cups	39	22
Soba noodles, instant, served in soup	46	1¼ cups	49	22
Udon noodles, cooked	62	1¼ cups	48	30
Nutella®, hazelnut spread Ⓖ	33	1 Tbsp.	12	4
Nutri-Grain™, breakfast cereal, Kellogg's®	66	½ cup	15	10
NUTS AND SEEDS				
Cashews, salted	22	1 ounce	9	2
Peanuts, roasted, salted	14	1.75 ounces	6	1

Food	GI	Nominal Serving Size	Available Carbs per Serving	GL per Serving
NUTS AND SEEDS (continued)				
Pecans, raw	10	1.75 ounces	3	1
Sesame seeds	★	2 Tbsp.	0.1	0
Oat bran and honey bread ⓖ	49	1 slice	13	7
Oat bran, unprocessed	55	2 Tbsp.	5	3
Oatmeal, instant, made with water	82	1 cup	26	17
Oatmeal, from old-fashioned oats, made with water	58	1 cup	21	11
Oatmeal, from steel-cut oats, made with water	52	1 cup	22	11
Oatmeal cookies, plain	54 ■	2 cookies (1 ounce)	17	9
Okra	★	½ cup	0	0
Onions	★	½ cup	0	0
Orange, fresh	42	1 small (4 ounces)	11	5
Orange juice, unsweetened	50	8 fluid ounces	18	9
Orange juice, unsweet-ened, from concentrate	53	8 fluid ounces	18	9
Oysters, plain, raw or cooked	★	3 ounces	0	0
Pancakes, 6", prepared from pancake mix	67 ■	1 pancake	23	15
Parsnips	97	½ cup	12	12
PASTA				
Capellini, white, boiled	45	1 cup	45	20
Cheese tortellini, cooked	50 ■	6 ounces	21	10
Corn pasta, gluten-free, cooked	78	1¼ cups	42	32
Fettuccine, egg noodles, cooked	40	1 cup	46	18

Food	GI	Nominal Serving Size	Available Carbs per Serving	GL per Serving
Gnocchi, cooked	68	6 ounces	48	33
Linguine, thick, durum wheat, cooked	46	1 cup	48	22
Linguine, thin, durum wheat, cooked	52	1 cup	45	23
Macaroni and cheese, Kraft®	64 ■	1¼ cups	51	32
Macaroni, white, durum wheat, cooked	47	1¼ cups	48	23
Macaroni, white, plain, cooked	47	1¼ cups	48	23
Ravioli, meat-filled, durum wheat flour, cooked	39 ■	6 ounces	38	15
Rice and corn pasta, gluten-free	76	1¼ cups	49	37
Rice pasta, brown, cooked	92	1 cup	38	35
Spaghetti, protein-enriched, cooked	27	1¼ cups	52	14
Spaghetti, white, durum wheat, cooked	44	1 cup	48	21
Spaghetti, wholewheat, cooked	42	1¼ cups	42	16
Spiral pasta, white, durum wheat, cooked	43	1¼ cups	44	19
Star Pastina, white, cooked	38	1 cup	48	18
Vermicelli, white, durum wheat, cooked	35	1 cup	44	16
Papaya, fresh	56	½ small (4 ounces)	8	5
Peach, fresh	42	1 medium (4 ounces)	11	5

Food	GI	Nominal Serving Size	Available Carbs per Serving	GL per Serving
Peaches, canned, in heavy syrup	58	½ cup	15	9
Peaches, canned, in light syrup	57	½ cup	18	9
Peaches, canned, in natural juice	45	½ cup	11	4
Peanuts, roasted, salted	14	1.75 ounces	6	1
Pear halves, canned, in natural juice	44	½ cup	13	5
Pear halves, canned, in light syrup	25	½ cup	14	4
Pear, fresh	38	1 medium (4 ounces)	11	4
Peas, green	48	½ cup	7	3
Pecan nuts, raw	10	1.75 ounces	3	1
Peppers	★	½ cup	0	0
Pineapple juice, unsweetened	46	8 fluid ounces	34	16
Pineapple, fresh	59	¾ cup	10	6
Pita bread, 4", white	57	1 pita	17	10
PIZZA				
Pizza, Super Supreme, pan, Pizza Hut	36 ■	3.5 ounces	24	9
Pizza, Super Supreme, thin and crispy, Pizza Hut	30 ■	3.5 ounces	22	7
Pizza, Vegetarian Supreme, thin and crispy, Pizza Hut	49 ■	7 ounces	50	25
Plum, raw	39	1 medium (4 ounces)	12	5
Polenta, cooked with water	68	⅔ cup	13	9
Pop-Tarts™, chocolate	70	1.75 ounces	36	25
Popcorn, plain, popped	72	2 cups	11	8

Food	GI	Nominal Serving Size	Available Carbs per Serving	GL per Serving
Pork	★ ■	3 ounces	0	0
Potato chips, plain, salted	54 ■	1.75 ounces	18	10
Potato crisps, plain, salted	54 ■	1.75 ounces	18	10
POTATOES				
French fries, frozen, reheated	75 ■	5 ounces	29	22
Potato, average, boiled	72	1 medium (5 ounces)	18	16
Potato, average, microwaved	79	1 medium (5 ounces)	18	14
Potato, russet, baked without fat	77	1 medium (5 ounces)	30	23
Potato, instant, mashed	88	¾ cup	20	18
Potato, new, canned	65	6 small (5 ounces)	18	12
Sweet potato, baked	46	1 medium (5 ounces)	25	11
Pound cake, plain, Sara Lee	54 ■	1 slice (1.75 ounces)	23	12
POULTRY				
Chicken, without the skin and bone	★ ■	3 ounces	0	0
Chicken nuggets, with breading, frozen, reheated	46 ■	3.5 ounces	16	7
Duck, without the skin and bone	★ ■	3 ounces	0	0
Turkey, without the skin and bone	★ ■	3 ounces	0	0
Power Bar®, chocolate	56	2 ounces	42	24
Pretzels, oven-baked, wheat flour	83	1 ounce	20	16
Prune juice, unsweetened	43	8 fluid ounces	30	13

Food	GI	Nominal Serving Size	Available Carbs per Serving	GL per Serving
Prunes, pitted, Sunsweet®	29	2 ounces	33	10
Pudding, chocolate, instant, package mix with whole milk	47	½ cup	16	7
Pudding, vanilla, instant, package mix with whole milk	40	½ cup	16	6
Puffed rice	80	2 cups	21	17
Puffed wheat	80	2 cups	21	17
Pumpernickel bread	50	1 slice	10	5
Pumpkin	75	½ cup	4	3
Pumpkin, creamy	76	8 fluid ounces	20	15
Quinoa, organic, boiled	53	¾ cup	17	9
Quick cooking brown rice, boiled	80	¾ cup	38	31
Radishes	★	½ cup	0	0
Raisin Bran™, breakfast cereal, Kellogg's®	73	½ cup	19	14
Raisin bread	63	1 slice	17	11
Raisins	64	2 ounces	44	28
Raspberries	★	½ cup	0	0
Ravioli, meat-filled, durum wheat flour, cooked	39 ■	6 ounces	38	15
Rhubarb	★	1 cup	0	0
RICE				
Arborio risotto rice, white, boiled	69	¾ cup	43	29
Basmati rice, white, boiled	58	1 cup	38	22
Brown rice, boiled	66	1 cup	37	24
Glutinous rice, white, cooked	98	¾ cup	32	31
Instant rice, white, boiled	87	¾ cup	42	29

Food	GI	Nominal Serving Size	Available Carbs per Serving	GL per Serving
Jasmine rice, white, long-grain, cooked	109	¾ cup	42	46
Long-grain rice, white, boiled	50	¾ cup	41	23
Quick cooking brown rice, boiled	80	¾ cup	38	31
Wild rice, boiled	57	¾ cup	32	18
Rice and corn pasta, gluten-free	76	1¼ cups	49	37
Rice bran, unprocessed	19	4 Tbsp.	14	3
Rice cakes, puffed, white	82	1 ounce	21	17
Rice Krispies®, breakfast cereal, Kellogg's®	82	1¼ cups	26	22
Rice Krispies Treat™ bar, Kellogg's®	63	1 ounce	24	15
Rice milk, average	92	8 fluid ounces	34	31
Rice milk, calcium-enriched Vitasoy®	79	8 fluid ounces	22	17
Rice pasta, brown, cooked	92	1 cup	38	35
Rice vermicelli, cooked	58	1¼ cups	39	22
Rich Tea Biscuits®	55 ■	1 ounce	19	10
Roll, dinner, white	73	1 small (1 ounce)	16	12
Roll-Ups®, processed fruit snack	99	1 ounce	25	24
Rye bread, black	76	1 slice	13	10
Rye bread, dark	86	1 slice	14	12
Rye bread, light	68	1 slice	14	10
Rye bread, seeded Ⓖ	51	1 slice	13	7
Ryvita® Original Rye crispbread	65	1 ounce	30	19
Ryvita® Sesame Original crispbread	64	1 ounce	28	18

Food	GI	Nominal Serving Size	Available Carbs per Serving	GL per Serving
Salami	★ ■	1 ounce	0	0
Salmon, canned in water	★	3 ounces	0	0
Sardines, canned	★	2 ounces	0	0
Scallops, plain, cooked	★	3 ounces	0	0
Scallions	★	2 Tbsp.	0	0
Scones, plain, made from package mix	92	1 ounce	9	8
SEAFOOD				
Calamari rings, squid, plain, without batter or bread crumbs	★	3 ounces	0	0
Clams, plain, steamed	★	3 ounces	0	0
Crabmeat, plain, without breading	★	3 ounces	0	0
Lobster, plain, cooked	★	3 ounces	0	0
Oysters, plain, raw or cooked	★	3 ounces	0	0
Scallops, plain, cooked	★	3 ounces	0	0
Shrimp, plain, cooked	★	3 ounces	0	0
Semolina, wheat, hot cereal, made with water	55	⅔ cup	11	6
Sesame seeds	★	2 Tbsp.	0.1	0
Shallots	★	2 Tbsp.	0	0
Shortbread cookies, plain	64 ■	2 cookies (1 ounce)	16	10
Shredded Wheat, breakfast cereal	75	½ cup	20	15
Shrimp, plain, cooked	★	3 ounces	0	0
Skittles®	70 ■	1.75 ounces	45	32
SNACK FOODS				
Apricot-filled fruit bar, made with whole grain flour	50 ■	1.75 ounces	34	17
Berry Bliss Nutrition Bar	22	1 bar	23	5

Food	GI	Nominal Serving Size	Available Carbs per Serving	GL per Serving
Cheese curls, cheese-flavored snack	74 ■	1.75 ounces	29	22
Chicken nuggets, frozen, reheated	46 ■	3.5 ounces	16	7
Chocolate Charger Nutrition Bar	28	1 bar	24	7
Chocolate hazelnut spread, Nutella® Ⓖ	30	1 Tbsp.	12	4
Corn chips, plain, salted	42 ■	1.75 ounces	25	11
Fish sticks	38 ■	3.5 ounces	19	7
French fries, frozen, reheated	75 ■	5 ounces	29	22
Gummi confectionery, made with glucose syrup	94	1.75 ounces	36	34
Jelly beans	78	1 ounce	28	22
Licorice, soft	78	2 ounces	42	33
Life Savers®, peppermint	70	1 ounce	30	21
M&M's®, peanut	33 ■	1 ounce	17	6
Mars Bar®, regular	62 ■	2 ounces	40	25
Marshmallows, plain, white	62	1 ounce	20	12
Mint Mania Nutrition Bar	23	1 bar	24	6
Muesli bar, chewy, with choc chips or fruit	54 ■	1 ounce	21	12
Muesli bar, crunchy, with dried fruit	61	1 ounce	21	13
Peanut Power Nutrition Bar	27	1 bar	22	6
Peanuts, roasted, salted	14	1.75 ounces	6	1
Pop-Tarts™, chocolate	70	1.75 ounces	36	25
Popcorn, plain, popped	72	2 cups	11	8
Potato chips, plain, salted	54 ■	1.75 ounces	18	10
Potato crisps, plain, salted	54 ■	1.75 ounces	18	10

Food	GI	Nominal Serving Size	Available Carbs per Serving	GL per Serving
SNACK FOODS (continued)				
Power Bar®, chocolate	56	2 ounces	42	24
Pretzels, oven-baked, wheat flour	83	1 ounce	20	16
Pudding, chocolate, instant, package mix, with whole milk	47 ■	½ cup	16	7
Pudding, vanilla, instant, package mix with whole milk	40	½ cup	16	6
Rice Krispies Treat™ bar, Kellogg's®	63	1 ounce	24	15
Roll-Ups®, processed fruit snack	99	1 ounce	25	24
Skittles®	70 ■	1.75 ounces	45	32
Snickers Bar®, regular	41 ■	2 ounces	36	15
Sushi, salmon	48	3.5 ounces	36	17
Twix® bar	44 ■	2 ounces	39	17
Waffles, plain	76 ■	1 ounce	13	10
Snowpea sprouts	★	½ cup	0	0
Snickers Bar®, regular	41 ■	2 ounces	36	15
Soba noodles, instant, served in soup	46	1¼ cups	49	22
SOFT DRINKS				
Soda, Coca-Cola®	53	8 fluid ounces	26	14
Soda, diet varieties	★	8 fluid ounces	0	0
Fanta®, orange soft drink	68	8 fluid ounces	34	23
SOUPS				
Black bean, canned	64	1 cup	27	17
Clear consommé, chicken or vegetable	★	8 fluid ounces	2	0

Food	GI	Nominal Serving Size	Available Carbs per Serving	GL per Serving
Green pea, canned	66	8 fluid ounces	41	27
Lentil, canned	44	8 fluid ounces	21	9
Minestrone, traditional	39	8 fluid ounces	18	7
Pumpkin, creamy	76	8 fluid ounces	20	15
Split pea, canned	60	8 fluid ounces	27	16
Tomato, canned	45	8 fluid ounces	17	6
Sourdough rye bread	48	1 slice	12	6
Sourdough wheat bread	54	1 slice	14	8
SOY				
Soy milk, full fat, calcium-fortified	36	8 fluid ounces	18	6
Soy milk, reduced-fat, calcium-fortified	44	8 fluid ounces	17	8
Soy smoothie drink, banana, low-fat	30	8 fluid ounces	22	7
Soy yogurt, fruited, 2% fat, with sugar	50	7 ounces	26	13
Soybeans, canned, drained	14	½ cup	6	1
Spaghetti, protein-enriched, cooked	27	1¼ cups	52	14
Spaghetti, white, durum wheat, cooked	44	1 cup	48	21
Spaghetti, wholewheat, cooked	42	1¼ cups	42	16
Special K®, breakfast cereal, Kellogg's®	56	1 cup	21	11
Spelt multigrain bread	54	1 slice	12	7
Spinach	★	1 cup	0	0

Food	GI	Nominal Serving Size	Available Carbs per Serving	GL per Serving
Spiral pasta, white, durum wheat, cooked	43	1¼ cups	44	19
Split pea soup, canned	60	8 fluid ounces	27	16
Sponge cake, plain, unfilled	46 ■	⅛ cake (2 ounces)	36	17
SPORTS DRINKS				
Gatorade®	78	8 fluid ounces	15	12
SPREADS				
Apricot fruit spread, reduced sugar	55	2 Tbsp.	13	7
Avocado	★	2 Tbsp.	0	0
Jam, Apricot, 100% fruit	50	1½ Tbsp	9	4.5
Jam, Blackberry, 100% fruit	46	1½ Tbsp	9	4
Jam, Raspberry, 100% fruit	46	1½ Tbsp	9	4
Jam, Strawberry, 100% fruit	46	1½ Tbsp	9	4
Diet jelly	★	2 Tbsp.	0	0
Golden syrup	63	1 Tbsp.	17	11
Honey, commercial-blend	64	1 Tbsp.	17	11
Honey, 100% pure floral	35	1 Tbsp.	18	6
Honey, various (averaged)	55	1 Tbsp.	18	10
Hummus, regular	6	2 Tbsp.	5	1
Maple flavored syrup	68	1 Tbsp.	22	15
Maple syrup, pure, Canadian	54	1 Tbsp	18	10
Marmalade, orange	55	1½ Tbsp.	20	9
Nutella® Ⓖ, hazelnut spread	33	1 Tbsp.	12	4
Squash, yellow	★	½ cup	0	0

Food	GI	Nominal Serving Size	Available Carbs per Serving	GL per Serving
Squid or calamari, without batter or bread crumbs	★	3 ounces	0	0
Star Pastina, white, cooked	38	1 cup	48	18
Steak, beef, lean	★ ■	3 ounces	0	0
Stoned Wheat Thins, crackers	67	1 ounce	17	12
Stoneground, 100% whole wheat bread	59	1 slice	12	7
Strawberries, fresh	40	1 cup	3	1
Stuffing, bread	74	½ cup	21	16
Sugar, granulated, white	68	1 Tbsp.	10	7
Sunflower and barley bread	57	1 slice	11	6
Sushi, salmon	48	3.5 ounces	36	17
Sweet corn, on the cob	48	1 medium ear	16	8
Sweet corn, whole kernel, canned, drained	46	⅓ cup	14	7
Sweet potato	46	1 medium (5 ounces)	25	11
Sweetened condensed full-fat milk	61 ■	2 fluid ounces	28	17
Swiss chard	★	1 cup	0	0
Taco shells, cornmeal-based, baked	68	.75 ounces	12	8
Taro	54	¼ cup	8	4
Tofu (bean curd), plain, unsweetened	★	3.5 ounces	0	0
Tomato	★	½ cup	0	0
Tomato juice, no added sugar	38	8 fluid ounces	9	4
Tomato soup, canned	45	8 fluid ounces	17	6
Tortellini, cheese, cooked	50 ■	6 ounces	21	10
Tortilla, wheat	30	1 medium (2 ounces)	26	8

Food	GI	Nominal Serving Size	Available Carbs per Serving	GL per Serving
Tortilla, wheat, with pinto beans and tomato sauce	28	3½ ounces	18	5
Tuna, canned in water	★	3 ounces	0	0
Turkey, without the skin and bone	★ ■	3 ounces	0	0
Turnip	★	½ cup	0	0
Twix® bar	44 ■	2 ounces	39	17
Udon noodles, plain, cooked	62	1¼ cups	48	30
Vanilla cake, cake mix with vanilla frosting, Betty Crocker	42 ■	1/12 cake (3.5 ounces)	58	24
Vanilla, custard, traditional, homemade	43 ■	½ cup	17	7
Vanilla, custard, reduced fat	37	½ cup	15	6
Vanilla pudding, instant, package mix with whole milk	40	½ cup	16	6
Vanilla wafer, plain	77 ■	7 small wafers (1 ounce)	18	14
Veal	★	3 ounces	0	0
VEGETABLES				
Alfalfa sprouts, raw	★	½ cup	0	0
Artichokes, globe, fresh or canned	★	½ cup	0	0
Arugula, raw	★	1 cup	0	0
Asparagus	★	½ cup	0	0
Bean sprouts	★	½ cup	0	0
Beets, red, canned	64	½ cup	7	5
Bok choy	★	½ cup	0	0
Broad beans (fava)	79	½ cup	11	9
Broccoli	★	½ cup	0	0

Food	GI	Nominal Serving Size	Available Carbs per Serving	GL per Serving
Brussels sprouts	★	½ cup	0	0
Cabbage	★	½ cup	0	0
Carrots, cooked	41	½ cup	5	2
Cauliflower	★	½ cup	0	0
Celery	★	½ cup	0	0
Chilies, fresh or dried	★	1 Tsp.	0	0
Chives, fresh	★	2 Tbsp.	0	0
Corn, sweet, on the cob	48	1 medium ear	16	8
Corn, sweet, whole kernel, canned	46	⅓ cup	14	7
Cucumber	★	½ cup	0	0
Eggplant	★	½ cup	0	0
Endive	★	1 cup	0	0
Fennel	★	½ cup	0	0
Garlic	★	1 clove	0	0
Ginger	★	1 Tsp.	0	0
Green beans	★	½ cup	0	0
Herbs, fresh or dried	★	2 Tbsp.	0	0
Leeks	★	½ cup	0	0
Lettuce	★	1 cup	0	0
Mushrooms	★	½ cup	0	0
Okra	★	½ cup	0	0
Onions	★	½ cup	0	0
Parsnips	97	½ cup	12	12
Peas, green	48	½ cup	7	3
Peppers	★	½ cup	0	0
Potato, average, boiled	72	1 medium (5 ounces)	18	16
Potato, average, microwaved	79	1 medium (5 ounces)	18	14
Potato, russet, baked without fat	85	1 medium (5 ounces)	30	26

Food	GI	Nominal Serving Size	Available Carbs per Serving	GL per Serving
VEGETABLES *(continued)*				
Potato, instant, mashed	85	¾ cup	20	17
Potato, new, canned	65	6 small (5 ounces)	18	12
Pumpkin	75	½ cup	4	3
Radishes	★	½ cup	0	0
Scallions	★	2 Tbsp.	0	0
Shallots	★	2 Tbsp.	0	0
Snowpea sprouts	★	½ cup	0	0
Spinach	★	1 cup	0	0
Squash, yellow	★	½ cup	0	0
Sweet potato	46	1 medium (5 ounces)	25	11
Swiss chard	★	1 cup	0	0
Taro	54	¼ cup	8	4
Tomato	★	½ cup	0	0
Turnip	★	½ cup	0	0
Watercress	★	1 cup	0	0
Yam	37	1 medium (5 ounces)	36	13
Zucchini	★	½ cup	0	0
Vermicelli, white, durum wheat, cooked	35	1 cup	44	16
Vinegar	★	2 Tbsp.	0	0
Waffles, plain	76 ■	1 ounce	13	10
Water crackers, plain	78	1 ounce	18	14
Watercress	★	1 cup	0	0
Watermelon	76	¾ cup	6	4
Weet-Bix, breakfast cereal, biscuits, regular	69	½ cup	17	12
White beans, cooked, canned	38	½ cup	31	12

Food	GI	Nominal Serving Size	Available Carbs per Serving	GL per Serving
White bread, enriched, sliced	71	1 slice	14	10
White chocolate, plain	44 ■	1.75 ounces	29	13
Whole wheat bread, made w/enriched wheat flour, sliced	71	1 slice	12	9
Whole wheat bread, 100%, stoneground	59	1 slice	12	7
Wild rice, boiled	57	¾ cup	32	18
Wonder White®, bread, sliced	80	1 slice	15	12
Yam	37	1 medium (5 ounces)	36	13
YOGURT				
Yogurt, fat-free, with sugar, French Vanilla	40	3.5 ounces	27	10
Yogurt, fat-free, with sugar, Mango	39	3.5 ounces	25	10
Yogurt, fat-free, with sugar, Strawberry	38	3.5 ounces	22	8
Yogurt, fat-free, with sugar, Wild Berry	38	3.5 ounces	22	8
Yogurt, fat-free, with sugar, average, various flavors	40	7 ounces	31	12
Yogurt, low-fat, no added sugar, vanilla or fruit	20	7 ounces	13	3
Yogurt, low-fat, with sugar, Apricot, Mango and Peach	26	3.5 ounces	15	4
Yogurt, low-fat, with sugar, French Vanilla	26	3.5 ounces	18	5
Yogurt, low-fat, with sugar, Wild Berry	28	3.5 ounces	15	4

Food	GI	Nominal Serving Size	Available Carbs per Serving	GL per Serving
Yogurt, low-fat, with sugar, Strawberry	28	3.5 ounces	15	4
Yogurt, soy, with sugar, average, fruited	50	7 ounces	26	13
Zucchini	★	½ cup	0	0

Low to High
GI Values

*T*hese tables are designed to enable you to make easy and effective substitutions to what you currently eat, to help you lower the GI of your diet as a whole.

> Low GI: 55 or under
> Medium GI: 56–69
> High GI: 70 or over

With this quick reference guide you can select the lower GI varieties in each food category. The foods are listed in three columns: low, medium, and high.

The food categories include:

Key

- ■ Means that a food may be high in saturated fat. As we have mentioned previously, the GI should not be used in isolation, but the overall nutritional value of the food needs to be considered.

- Ⓖ Means that a food has been accurately tested for its GI and meets strict nutritional criteria. You can be assured that these foods are healthier choices within their food group.

APPLE JUICE

Low	Medium	High
Apple and black-currant juice, unsweetened		
Apple and cherry juice, unsweetened Ⓖ		
Apple and mango juice, unsweetened Ⓖ		
Apple juice, clear, no added sugar Ⓖ		
Apple juice, cloudy, no added sugar Ⓖ		

BEANS/LEGUMES

Low	Medium	High
Baked beans, canned in tomato sauce, Heinz®		
Black beans, boiled		
Black-eyed peas, boiled		
Butter beans, boiled		
Cannellini beans, canned		
Chickpeas, canned		
Kidney beans, dark red, canned, drained		
Kidney beans, red, canned, drained		
Lentils, green or brown, dried, boiled		
Lentils, red, dried, boiled		
Lima beans, baby, frozen, reheated		
Mung beans		
Soybeans, canned, drained		
Split peas, yellow, boiled		
White beans, canned		

BEVERAGES

Low	Medium	High
Coffee, black, no milk or sugar	Fanta®, orange soft drink	Gatorade®
Ensure™, vanilla, nutritional supplement		
Malted milk powder in reduced-fat milk		
Malted milk powder in skim milk		
Malted milk powder in whole milk ■		
Nestle Quik® powder, Chocolate, in reduced-fat milk		
Nestle Quik® powder, Strawberry, in reduced-fat milk		
Slim-Fast® drink, can, vanilla or chocolate		
Slim-Fast® drink powder, all flavors, made with skim milk		
Soda, Coca-Cola®		
Soda, diet varieties		

BREAD

Low	Medium	High
9 Grain multigrain bread Ⓖ	Hamburger bun, white	Bagel, white
Flaxseed and soy bread	Pita bread, 4", white	Dinner roll, white
Oat bran and honey bread Ⓖ	Raisin bread	Gluten-free, multi-grain bread
Pumpernickel bread	Rye bread, light	Kaiser roll, white
Sourdough rye bread	Rye bread, seeded Ⓖ	Rye bread, black
Sourdough wheat bread	Sunflower and barley bread	Rye bread, dark
Spelt multigrain bread	Whole wheat bread, 100%, stoneground	Stuffing, bread
Tortilla, wheat		White bread, enriched, sliced
		Whole wheat bread, made w/ enriched wheat flour, sliced
		Wonder White®, bread, sliced

BREAKFAST CEREALS

Low	Medium	High
All-Bran®, Kellogg's®	Froot Loops®, Kellogg's®	Bran Flakes, Kellogg's®
Frosted Flakes®, Kellogg's®	Just Right®, Kellogg's®	Coco Pops®, Kellogg's®
Oat bran, raw, unprocessed	Muesli, Swiss Formula	Corn Flakes®, Kellogg's®
Oatmeal, from steel-cut oats, made with water	Nutri-Grain™, Kellogg's®	Corn Pops®, Kellogg's®
Muesli, natural	Oatmeal, from old-fashioned oats, made with water	Crispix®
Muesli, toasted	Special K®, Kellogg's®	Honey Smacks®, Kellogg's®
Rice bran, unprocessed	Weet-Bix, biscuits, regular	Oatmeal, instant, made with water
Semolina, wheat, hot cereal, made with water		Puffed wheat
		Rice Krispies®, Kellogg's®
		Puffed rice
		Raisin Bran™, Kellogg's®
		Shredded Wheat

CAKES

Low	Medium	High
Chocolate cake, cake mix with frosting, Betty Crocker ■	Angel food cake, plain ■	Cupcake with strawberry icing ■
Banana bread, homemade ■		
Pound cake, plain, Sara Lee ■		
Sponge cake, plain, unfilled ■		
Vanilla cake, cake mix with vanilla frosting, Betty Crocker ■		

CEREAL GRAINS

Low	Medium	High
Barley, pearled, boiled	Cornmeal (polenta), cooked with water	Millet, boiled
Buckwheat, groats, boiled	Couscous, boiled	
Bulgur, cracked wheat, ready to eat		
Quinoa, organic, boiled		

CHOCOLATE

Low	Medium	High
Cadbury's® Milk Chocolate, plain ■	Mars Bar®, regular ■	
Chocolate cake, cake mix with frosting, Betty Crocker ■		
Chocolate pudding, instant, package mix, with whole milk ■		
Dark chocolate, plain ■		
Dove®, milk chocolate ■		
M&M's®, peanut ■		
Milk chocolate, plain, with fructose instead of sugar ■		
Nestle®, milk chocolate bar		
Snickers Bar®, regular ■		
Twix® bar ■		
White chocolate, plain ■		

COOKIES

Low	Medium	High
Oatmeal cookies, plain ■	Arrowroot biscuits ■	Graham crackers, plain ■
Rich Tea Biscuits® ■	Digestives®, cookies, plain ■	Vanilla wafer, plain ■
	Shortbread, plain ■	

CRACKERS AND CRISPBREADS

Low	Medium	High
	Ryvita® Original Rye crispbread	Rice cakes, white
	Ryvita® Sesame Original crispbread	Water crackers, plain
	Stoned Wheat Thins®	Melba toast, plain

FISH

Low	Medium	High
Fish, all-types, fresh or frozen, without skin		
Fish sticks, lightly breaded ■		
Salmon, canned in water		
Sardines, canned		
Tuna, canned in water		

FRUIT AND VEGETABLE JUICE

Low	Medium	High
Apple and blackcurrant, unsweetened		
Apple and cherry, unsweetened Ⓖ		
Apple and mango, unsweetened Ⓖ		
Apple juice, clear, no added sugar Ⓖ		
Apple juice, cloudy, no added sugar Ⓖ		
Carrot, freshly made		
Cranberry Juice Cocktail, Ocean Spray®		
Grapefruit, unsweetened		
Orange, unsweetened, fresh		
Orange, unsweetened, from concentrate		
Pineapple, unsweetened		
Prune, unsweetened		
Tomato, no added sugar		

FRUIT, CANNED

Low	Medium	High
Fruit cocktail, in natural juice	Apricots, in light syrup	Lychees, in syrup, drained
Peaches, in natural juice	Peaches, in light syrup	
Pear halves, in light syrup	Peaches, in heavy syrup	
Pears, in natural juice		

FRUIT, DRIED

Low	Medium	High
Apple	Cranberries, sweetened	Dates, pitted
Apricots	Figs, dried	
Prunes, pitted, Sunsweet®	Raisins	

FRUIT, FRESH

Low	Medium	High
Apple	Apricots	Watermelon
Banana, ripe	Cherries, dark	
Custard apple	Canteloupe	
Grapefruit	Papaya	
Grapes	Pineapple	
Kiwi fruit		
Lemon		
Lime		
Mango		
Montmorency Frozen Tart Cherries		
Orange		
Peach		
Pear		
Plum		
Raspberries		
Rhubarb		
Strawberries		

GLUTEN-FREE PRODUCTS

Low	Medium	High
		Gluten-free buckwheat pancakes, 6", from pancake mix
		Gluten-free corn pasta, cooked
		Gluten-free multigrain bread
		Gluten-free rice and corn pasta, cooked

ICE CREAM

Low	Medium	High
Gelati, sugar-free, chocolate		
Gelati, sugar-free, vanilla		
Ice cream, full-fat, chocolate ■		
Ice cream, low-fat, chocolate Ⓖ		
Ice cream, low-fat, vanilla Ⓖ		
Ice cream, full-fat, vanilla ■		

MEAT

Low	Medium	High
Bacon, lean		
Beef, ground, lean ■		
Beef pot pie, with crust ■		
Beef, steak, lean ■		
Ham, lean ■		
Lamb, lean		
Pork ■		
Salami ■		
Chicken, without the skin and bone ■		
Chicken nuggets, with breading, frozen, reheated ■		
Duck, without the skin and bone ■		
Turkey, without the skin and bone ■		
Veal		

MILK

Low	Medium	High
Milk, 1%, light, low-fat	Condensed milk, sweetened, full-fat ■	Rice milk, average
Milk, 2%, reduced-fat		
Milk, fat-free, skim, nonfat		
Milk, whole, full-fat ■		
Milk, low-fat, chocolate, with aspartame		
Milk, low-fat, chocolate, with sugar		
Rice milk, calcium-enriched Vitasoy®		
Soy milk, full-fat, calcium-fortified		
Soy milk, reduced-fat, calcium-fortified		

MUFFINS

Low	Medium	High
Apple muffin, homemade ■	Blueberry muffin, commercially-made ■	
	Bran muffin, commercially-made ■	
	Carrot muffin, commercially-made ■	

NOODLES

Low	Medium	High
Mung bean noodles, cooked	Instant noodles, 99% fat free, dry, package	
Soba noodles, instant, served in soup	Rice vermicelli, cooked	
	Udon noodles, cooked	

NUTS AND SEEDS

Low	Medium	High
Cashews, salted		
Peanuts, roasted, salted		
Pecans, raw		
Sesame seeds		

PASTA

Low	Medium	High
Cheese tortellini, cooked ■	Gnocchi, cooked	Corn pasta, gluten-free, cooked
Fettuccine, egg noodles, cooked	Macaroni and cheese, Kraft® ■	Ravioli, meat-filled, durum wheat flour, cooked ■
Macaroni, white, durum wheat, cooked		Rice and corn pasta, gluten-free
Macaroni, white, plain, cooked		Rice pasta, brown, cooked
Capellini, white, boiled		
Linguine, thick, durum wheat, cooked		
Macaroni, white, durum wheat, cooked		
Macaroni, white, plain, cooked		
Spaghetti, protein-enriched, cooked		
Spaghetti, white, durum wheat, cooked		
Spaghetti, whole-wheat, cooked		
Spiral pasta, white, durum wheat, cooked		

PASTA *(continued)*

Low	Medium	High
Spaghetti, protein-enriched, cooked		
Star Pastina, white, cooked		
Vermicelli, white, durum wheat, cooked		

PIZZA

Low	Medium	High
Pizza, Super Supreme, pan, Pizza Hut ■		
Pizza, Super Supreme, thin and crispy, Pizza Hut ■		
Pizza, Vegetarian Supreme, thin and crispy, Pizza Hut ■		

POTATOES

Low	Medium	High
Sweet potato, baked	Potato, new, canned	French fries, frozen, reheated ■
		Potato, average, boiled
		Potato, average, microwaved
		Potato, instant, mashed
		Potato, russet, baked without fat

RICE

Low	Medium	High
Long-grain rice, white, boiled	Arborio risotto rice, white, boiled	Glutinous rice, white, cooked
	Basmati rice, white, boiled	Instant rice, white, boiled
	Brown rice, boiled	Jasmine rice, white, long-grain, cooked
	Wild rice, boiled	Quick cooking brown rice, boiled

SEAFOOD

Low	Medium	High
Calamari rings, squid, plain, without batter or bread crumbs		
Clams, plain, steamed		
Crabmeat, plain, without breading		
Lobster, plain, cooked		
Oysters, plain, raw or cooked		
Scallops, plain, cooked		
Shrimp, plain, cooked		

SNACK FOODS

Low	Medium	High
Apricot-filled fruit bar, made with whole grain flour ■	Mars Bar®, regular ■	Cheese curls, cheese-flavored snack ■
Berry Bliss Nutrition Bar	Muesli bar, crunchy, with dried fruit	French fries, frozen, reheated ■
Chicken nuggets, frozen, reheated ■	Power Bar®, chocolate	Gummi confectionery, made with glucose syrup
Choclate Charger Nutrition Bar	Rice Krispies Treat™ bar, Kellogg's®	Jelly beans
Chocolate hazelnut spread. Nutella® Ⓖ		Licorice, soft
Corn chips, plain, salted ■		Life Savers®, peppermint
Fish sticks ■		Pop-Tarts™, chocolate
M&M's®, peanut ■		Popcorn, plain, popped
Marshmallows, plain, white		Pretzels, ovenbaked, wheat flour
Mint Mania Nutrition Bar		Roll-Ups®, processed fruit snack
Muesli bar, chewy, with choc chips or fruit ■		Skittles® ■
Peanut Power Nutrition Bar		Waffles, plain ■
Peanuts, roasted, salted		
Potato chips, plain, salted ■		

SNACK FOODS *(continued)*

Low	Medium	High
Potato crisps, plain, salted ■		
Pudding, chocolate, instant, package mix, with whole milk ■		
Pudding, vanilla, instant, package mix with whole milk		
Snickers Bar®, regular ■		
Sushi, salmon		
Twix® bar ■		

SOUPS

Low	Medium	High
Clear consommé, chicken or vegetable	Black bean, canned	
Lentil, canned	Green pea, canned	
Minestrone, traditional	Pumpkin, creamy	
Tomato, canned	Split pea, canned	

SOY

Low	Medium	High
Soybeans, canned, drained		
Soy milk, full-fat, calcium-fortified		
Soy milk, reduced fat, calcium-fortified		
Soy smoothie drink, banana, low-fat		
Soy yogurt, fruited, 2% fat, with sugar		

SPREADS

Low	Medium	High
Apricot fruit spread, reduced sugar	Golden syrup	
Avocado	Honey, commercial-blend	
Diet jelly	Hummus, regular	
Jam, Apricot, 100% fruit	Maple flavored syrup	
Jam, Blackberry, 100% fruit		
Jam, Raspberry, 100% fruit		
Jam, Strawberry, 100% fruit		
Honey, 100% pure floral		
Honey, various (averaged)		
Maple syrup, pure, Canadian		
Marmalade, orange		
Nutella® ⓖ, hazelnut spread		

VEGETABLES

Low	Medium	High
Alfalfa sprouts, raw	Beets, red, canned	Broad beans (fava)
Artichokes, globe, fresh or canned	Potato, new, canned	Parsnips
Arugula, raw		Potato, average, boiled
Asparagus		Potato, average, microwaved
Bean sprouts		Potato, instant, mashed
Bok choy		Potato, russet, baked without fat
Broccoli		Pumpkin
Brussels sprouts		
Cabbage		
Carrots, cooked		
Cauliflower		
Celery		
Chillies, fresh or dried		
Chives, fresh		
Corn, sweet, on the cob		
Corn, sweet, whole kernel, canned		
Cucumber		
Eggplant		
Endive		
Fennel		
Garlic		
Ginger		
Green beans		
Leeks		

VEGETABLES *(continued)*

Low	Medium	High
Lettuce		
Mushrooms		
Okra		
Onions		
Peas, green		
Peppers		
Radishes		
Scallions		
Shallots		
Snowpea sprouts		
Spinach		
Squash, yellow		
Sweet potato		
Swiss chard		
Taro		
Tomato		
Turnip		
Watercress		
Yam		
Zucchini		

YOGURT

Low	Medium	High
Yogurt, fat-free, with sugar, French Vanilla		
Yogurt, fat-free, with sugar, Mango		
Yogurt, fat-free, with sugar, Strawberry		
Yogurt, fat-free, with sugar, Wild Berry		
Yogurt, fat-free, with sugar, average, various flavors		
Yogurt, low-fat, no added sugar, vanilla or fruit		
Yogurt, low-fat, with sugar, Apricot, Mango and Peach		
Yogurt, low-fat, with sugar, French Vanilla		
Yogurt, low-fat, with sugar, Wild Berry		
Yogurt, low-fat, with sugar, Strawberry		
Yogurt, soy, with sugar, average, fruited		